Colostomy ileostomy ostomy program for beginners

A new 3 in 1 delicious solution recipes program that pursue and cure all the pain, including healthy and appetizer recipes to stay fitness.

Dr. D. SAM

TABLE OF CONTENT

INTRODUCTION

"Welcome to a new chapter in your life! Our Colostomy, Ileostomy, and Ostomy Program for Beginners is your trusted companion on the journey to mastering your ostomy care. With empathy, expertise, and encouragement, we'll guide you through the essentials of ostomy management, lifestyle adjustments, and emotional well-being. Embrace your new normal and regain control, confidence, and freedom. Start your journey today!"

Chapter 1:DESCRIBE COLONOSTOMY, ILEOSTOMY, AND OSTOMY.

The phrases "ostomy," "ileostomy," and "colostomy" all refer to various surgically made apertures or diversions in the human body intended to facilitate the removal of waste.

Colostomy: A colostomy is a surgical technique in which a stoma, or opening, is created by bringing a section of the colon (large intestine) through the abdominal wall. Stool and other waste products are directed via this stoma and into a bag that is fastened to the abdomen, avoiding the rectum and anus. Colostomies are commonly carried out in patients with inflammatory bowel disorders, colorectal cancer, or other disorders affecting the lower colon or rectum.

Ileostomy: An ileostomy is a surgical operation where a stoma is created by bringing the terminal piece of the ileum—the last segment of the small intestine—through the abdominal wall. This stoma allows digestive waste to exit into an external bag or pouch. When the entire colon needs to be removed, ileostomies are frequently performed in patients with ulcerative colitis, Crohn's disease, or other disorders affecting the colon or rectum.

Ostomy: This is a generic term that includes several forms of surgically made holes or diversions, including ileostomy and colostomy. It describes any surgical operation that makes a stoma, or artificial opening, in the body to allow waste products to be expelled. When referring to any kind of surgically induced diversion, including colostomies, ileostomies, urostomies (for urine diversion), and other varieties, the term "ostomy" is sometimes used as a catch-all.

To collect the waste that travels through the stoma, people with ostomies wear special ostomy pouches or bags. These operations are usually carried out when an organ, wound, or other medical condition requires the bypassing of a section of the digestive or urinary system.

Edit To prevent complications and preserve correct ostomy function, some foods may need to be avoided or limited for people with a colostomy, ileostomy, or any other type of ostomy. The following are broad recommendations on foods to stay away from:

High-fiber foods: High-fiber foods can be difficult to digest and may raise the risk of obstruction or create blockages. Examples of such foods are raw fruits and vegetables with skins, nuts, seeds, whole grains, and bran. It is best to introduce these meals gradually and in modest portions.

Foods that produce gas: Beans, broccoli, cabbage, cauliflower, and carbonated drinks are among the foods that are known to produce gas and can lead to bloating, discomfort, and excessive gas production.

Foods that are spicy and high in fat: Foods that are spicy, fried, or fatty might irritate the digestive tract and result in cramps or diarrhea.

Beer and caffeinated drinks: These include coffee, tea, and sodas. They can also function as diuretics, which can cause dehydration and raise the risk of diarrhea and upset stomach.

Meats that are tough or fibrous: Meats that are tough or fibrous, such steak or pork chops, can be harder to digest and raise the possibility of blockages or obstructions.

Fried and sugary foods: Consuming a lot of sugar and fried foods might lead to dehydration and induce frequent bowel motions.

Foods that are hard to digest, such popcorn, nuts, and seeds, might impede or cause blockages in the ostomy.

It's crucial to remember that everyone has a varied tolerance for different foods, and figuring out which things you can eat most comfortably may need some trial and error.

A certified dietician or healthcare expert should be consulted for individualized dietary advice based on the kind of ostomy and the needs of the individual.

Chapter 3:WHAT FOODS ARE GENERALLY RECOMMENDED FOR PEOPLE WITH COLOSTOMY ILEOSTOMY OSTOMY?

Certain meals are often advised to help maintain optimal ostomy function and overall health for those with a colostomy, ileostomy, or any sort of ostomy. The following are some broad recommendations for things to eat:

lacking-fiber foods: Foods lacking in fiber are easier to digest and less prone to induce blockages or obstructions. Examples of such foods include white bread, white rice, pasta, and peeled fruits and vegetables. Foods high in protein: Fish, poultry, eggs, low-fat dairy products, lean meats, and poultry are all great sources of protein, which is necessary for both healing and general health maintenance.

Cooked veggies: In general, people can tolerate cooked veggies better than raw ones. Examples of this include carrots, squash, and green beans.

Bananas: They can thicken the consistency of the ostomy output and are a rich source of potassium.

Fruit juices and applesauce: These can supplement a diet lacking in moisture and may be more easily digested than entire fruits.

Probiotics: Foods high in probiotics, such kefir and yogurt, can improve digestion by supporting a balanced gut flora.

Consuming oral hydration solutions, like sports drinks or electrolyte-rich drinks, can assist in replenishing lost electrolytes and fluids.

Low-fiber, soft cereals: Oatmeal and cream of wheat are examples of low-fiber, soft cereals that can be a rich source of carbohydrates and may be easier to digest than high-fiber cereals.

It's crucial to remember that everyone has a varied tolerance for different meals, and figuring out which ones you can eat most comfortably may take some time. It is advised to begin with a low-fiber diet and add new foods gradually while monitoring any negative reactions. A trained dietitian or other healthcare provider should be consulted for individualized dietary advice based on the kind of ostomy and the needs of the individual.

Chapter 4:BREAKFAST RECIPES

Smooth Oatmeal

Ingredients:
- 1 cup old-fashioned oats
- 2 cups low-fat milk or non-dairy milk
- 1/4 teaspoon salt
- 1 teaspoon sugar or honey (optional)

- 1/2 cup blueberries or sliced bananas (optional)

Instructions:

1. In a saucepan, combine the oats, milk, and salt.
2. Bring the mixture to a boil over medium heat, stirring frequently.
3. Reduce the heat to low and cook for 5-7 minutes, stirring occasionally, until the oatmeal reaches your desired consistency.
4. Remove from heat and stir in sugar or honey, if desired.
5. Top with blueberries or sliced bananas (optional).

Egg White Omelet

Ingredients:

- 4 egg whites
- 1/4 cup low-fat shredded cheddar cheese
- 1/4 cup diced cooked turkey or chicken (optional)
- Salt and pepper to taste

Instructions:

1. Whisk the egg whites in a small bowl until frothy.
2. Spray a non-stick skillet with cooking spray and heat over medium heat.
3. Pour the egg whites into the skillet and let them cook for a minute or two.
4. Use a spatula to gently lift the edges of the omelet, allowing the uncooked egg to flow underneath.
5. When the omelet is nearly set, sprinkle the cheese and cooked turkey or chicken (if using) over one half of the omelet.
6. Fold the other half of the omelet over the filling.
7. Slide the omelet onto a plate and season with salt and pepper to taste.

Creamy Rice Pudding

Ingredients:

- 1 cup cooked white rice
- 2 cups low-fat milk
- 1/4 cup sugar

- 1 teaspoon vanilla extract
- 1/4 teaspoon ground cinnamon

Instructions:

1. In a saucepan, combine the cooked rice, milk, sugar, and vanilla extract.
2. Bring the mixture to a simmer over medium heat, stirring frequently.
3. Reduce the heat to low and cook for 15-20 minutes, stirring occasionally, until the mixture thickens to your desired consistency.
4. Remove from heat and stir in the ground cinnamon.
5. Serve warm or chilled.

Avocado Toast

Ingredients:

- 2 slices of white bread or sourdough bread
- 1 ripe avocado, mashed
- 1 teaspoon lemon juice
- Salt and pepper to taste
- Sliced tomatoes or cucumber (optional)

Instructions:
1. Toast the bread slices.
2. In a small bowl, mash the avocado and mix it with the lemon juice, salt, and pepper.
3. Spread the mashed avocado mixture evenly over the toasted bread slices.
4. Top with sliced tomatoes or cucumber (optional).

Applesauce Pancakes

Ingredients:
- 1 cup all-purpose flour
- 2 teaspoons baking powder
- 1/4 teaspoon salt
- 1 egg
- 1 cup low-fat milk
- 1/2 cup unsweetened applesauce
- 1 tablespoon vegetable oil or melted butter

Instructions
1. In a large bowl, whisk together the flour, baking powder, and salt.

2. In a separate bowl, beat the egg, then whisk in the milk, applesauce, and vegetable oil or melted butter.
3. Pour the wet ingredients into the dry ingredients and whisk until just combined (do not overmix).
4. Heat a non-stick skillet or griddle over medium heat.
5. Pour the batter onto the hot surface, using about 1/4 cup for each pancake.
6. Cook until bubbles appear on the surface, then flip and cook until golden brown on both sides.
7. Serve warm with a drizzle of maple syrup or honey (optional).

Scrambled Egg Whites with Spinach

Ingredients:
- 4 egg whites
- 1 cup fresh spinach, chopped
- 1 tablespoon low-fat milk
- Salt and pepper to taste
- 1 tablespoon grated Parmesan cheese (optional)

Instructions:

1. Whisk the egg whites and milk together in a small bowl.
2. Spray a non-stick skillet with cooking spray and heat over medium heat.
3. Add the chopped spinach to the skillet and cook for 1-2 minutes until wilted.
4. Pour in the egg white mixture and season with salt and pepper.
5. Use a spatula to gently scramble the eggs, stirring occasionally, until cooked to your desired doneness.
6. Sprinkle with Parmesan cheese (optional) before serving.

Baked Banana Oatmeal Cups

Ingredients:
- 2 ripe bananas, mashed
- 1 1/2 cups old-fashioned oats
- 1 cup low-fat milk or non-dairy milk
- 1 egg
- 1 teaspoon baking powder
- 1/2 teaspoon vanilla extract
- 1/4 teaspoon ground cinnamon

Instructions:
1. Preheat the oven to 350°F (175°C).
2. In a bowl, mix together the mashed bananas, oats, milk, egg, baking powder, vanilla extract, and cinnamon until well combined.
3. Grease a muffin tin or use silicone muffin cups.
4. Spoon the oatmeal mixture into the prepared muffin cups, filling them about 3/4 full.
5. Bake for 20-25 minutes, or until the oatmeal cups are set and slightly golden on top.
6. Let cool for a few minutes before serving.

Cottage Cheese and Fruit Parfait

Ingredients:
- 1 cup low-fat cottage cheese
- 1 cup diced peeled peaches or pears
- (fresh or canned in water)
- 1/4 cup low-fat granola or crushed graham crackers

Instructions

1. In a bowl or parfait glass, layer half of the cottage cheese, then half of the diced fruit.
2. Sprinkle with half of the granola or crushed graham crackers.
3. Repeat the layers with the remaining cottage cheese, fruit, and granola or crushed graham crackers.
4. Serve chilled.

Vegetable and Egg White Frittata

Ingredients:
- 8 egg whites
- 1/2 cup diced cooked potatoes
- 1/2 cup diced bell peppers
- 1/4 cup diced onions
- Salt and pepper to taste
- 1 tablespoon grated low-fat cheddar cheese (optional)

Instructions:

1. Preheat the oven to 350°F (175°C).
2. Whisk the egg whites in a bowl and season with salt and pepper.

3. Spray a non-stick oven-safe skillet or baking dish with cooking spray.
4. Add the diced potatoes, bell peppers, and onions to the skillet or baking dish and spread evenly.
5. Pour the egg white mixture over the vegetables.
6. Bake for 20-25 minutes, or until the frittata is set and cooked through.
7. Sprinkle with grated cheddar cheese (optional) before serving.

Smoothie Bowl

Ingredients:
- 1 cup low-fat milk or non-dairy milk
- 1/2 cup low-fat plain Greek yogurt
- 1 ripe banana
- 1/2 cup fresh or frozen berries
- 1 tablespoon honey or maple syrup (optional)
- Toppings: sliced bananas, granola, chia seeds, etc.

Instructions:

1. In a blender, combine the milk, yogurt, banana, berries, and honey or maple syrup (if using).
2. Blend until smooth and creamy.
3. Pour the smoothie mixture into a bowl.
4. Top with sliced bananas, granola, chia seeds, or other desired toppings.

Chapter 5: LUNCH RECIPES

Creamy Chicken and Rice Soup

Ingredients:
- 1 boneless, skinless chicken breast, cooked and shredded
- 4 cups low-sodium chicken broth
- 1 cup cooked white rice
- 1/2 cup sliced carrots
- 1/4 cup all-purpose flour
- 1/4 cup low-fat milk
- Salt and pepper to taste

Instructions:

1. In a saucepan, combine the chicken broth, shredded chicken, carrots, and cooked rice.
2. In a separate bowl, whisk together the flour and milk until smooth.
3. Slowly pour the flour-milk mixture into the saucepan, whisking constantly.
4. Bring the mixture to a simmer and cook for 5-7 minutes, or until thickened to your desired consistency.
5. Season with salt and pepper to taste.

Tuna Salad Sandwich

Ingredients:
- 1 (5 oz) can tuna, drained
- 2 tablespoons low-fat mayonnaise
- 1 tablespoon diced celery
- 1 tablespoon diced red onion (optional)
- Salt and pepper to taste
- 2 slices white bread or sourdough bread

Instructions:

1. In a bowl, combine the tuna, mayonnaise, celery, and red onion (if using).
2. Season with salt and pepper to taste and mix well.
3. Spread the tuna salad mixture evenly onto one slice of bread.
4. Top with the other slice of bread.

Egg Salad Lettuce Wraps

Ingredients:
- 4 hard-boiled eggs, chopped
- 2 tablespoons low-fat mayonnaise
- 1 tablespoon diced celery
- 1 tablespoon diced red onion (optional)
- Salt and pepper to taste
- 4 large lettuce leaves (e.g., romaine, iceberg, or butter lettuce)

Instructions:
1. In a bowl, combine the chopped hard-boiled eggs, mayonnaise, celery, and red onion (if using).

2. Season with salt and pepper to taste and mix well.
3. Scoop the egg salad mixture onto the lettuce leaves.
4. Wrap the lettuce leaves around the egg salad to form a handheld wrap.

Vegetable and Tofu Stir-Fry

Ingredients:
- 1 tablespoon vegetable oil
- 1 cup diced firm tofu
- 1 cup sliced mushrooms
- 1 cup sliced bell peppers
- 1 cup sliced zucchini
- 2 tablespoons low-sodium soy sauce or tamari
- Salt and pepper to taste
- Cooked white rice or quinoa (optional)

Instructions:
1. Heat the vegetable oil in a large skillet or wok over medium-high heat.
2. Add the diced tofu and stir-fry for 2-3 minutes until lightly browned.

3. Add the sliced mushrooms, bell peppers, and zucchini to the skillet.
4. Stir-fry for 5-7 minutes, or until the vegetables are tender-crisp.
5. Add the soy sauce or tamari and stir to combine.
6. Season with salt and pepper to taste.
7. Serve over cooked white rice or quinoa (optional).

Grilled Cheese and Tomato Soup

Ingredients:
- 4 slices white bread
- 4 slices low-fat cheddar cheese
- 2 tablespoons butter or margarine
- 1 (14 oz) can low-sodium tomato soup
- 1/2 cup low-fat milk

Instructions:
1. Preheat a skillet or griddle over medium heat.
2. For each sandwich, place two slices of bread and two slices of cheese between them.

3. Spread a thin layer of butter or margarine on the outsides of the sandwiches.
4. Cook the sandwiches in the preheated skillet or griddle until the bread is golden brown and the cheese is melted, about 2-3 minutes per side.
5. In a saucepan, combine the tomato soup and milk. Heat over medium heat, stirring occasionally, until heated through but not boiling.
6. Serve the grilled cheese sandwiches with the tomato soup on the side.

Baked Potato with Toppings

Ingredients:
- 2 medium russet potatoes
- 2 tablespoons low-fat sour cream
- 2 tablespoons diced cooked chicken or turkey
- 2 tablespoons shredded low-fat cheddar cheese
- 2 tablespoons diced tomatoes
- 2 tablespoons sliced green onions

- Salt and pepper to taste

Instructions:

1. Preheat the oven to 400°F (200°C).
2. Scrub the potatoes clean and prick them several times with a fork.
3. Bake the potatoes directly on the oven rack for 50-60 minutes, or until they are tender when pierced with a fork.
4. Remove the potatoes from the oven and let them cool slightly.
5. Cut each potato in half lengthwise and fluff the insides with a fork.
6. Top each potato half with sour cream, diced cooked chicken or turkey, shredded cheese, diced tomatoes, and sliced green onions.
7. Season with salt and pepper to taste.

Quinoa and Vegetable Salad

Ingredients:

- 1 cup cooked quinoa
- 1/2 cup diced cucumber
- 1/2 cup diced tomatoes
- 1/4 cup diced red onion

- 2 tablespoons chopped fresh parsley
- 2 tablespoons olive oil
- 1 tablespoon lemon juice
- Salt and pepper to taste

Instructions:

1. In a large bowl, combine the cooked quinoa, diced cucumber, tomatoes, red onion, and chopped parsley.
2. In a small bowl, whisk together the olive oil and lemon juice.
3. Pour the olive oil-lemon dressing over the quinoa and vegetable mixture and toss gently to combine.
4. Season with salt and pepper to taste.

Hummus and Vegetable Wrap

Ingredients:

- 2 large whole-wheat or low-fiber tortillas
- 1/2 cup hummus
- 1/2 cup sliced cucumber
- 1/2 cup sliced bell peppers
- 1/4 cup sliced red onion

- 2 tablespoons crumbled feta cheese (optional)

Instructions:
1. Spread half of the hummus evenly over each tortilla.
2. Top one half of each tortilla with sliced cucumber, bell peppers, and red onion.
3. Sprinkle with crumbled feta cheese (if using).
4. Fold the other half of the tortilla over the filling to form a wrap.

Turkey and Avocado Sandwich

Ingredients:
- 4 slices white or sourdough bread
- 4 oz sliced deli turkey
- 1 ripe avocado, mashed
- 2 tablespoons low-fat mayonnaise
- 1 tomato, sliced
- Lettuce leaves

Instructions:
1. Toast the bread slices, if desired.

2. In a small bowl, combine the mashed avocado and low-fat mayonnaise.
3. Spread the avocado mixture evenly on two slices of bread.
4. Top the avocado spread with sliced deli turkey, tomato slices, and lettuce leaves.
5. Top with the remaining two slices of bread.

Lentil and Sweet Potato Soup

Ingredients:
- 1 cup cooked lentils
- 1 cup diced cooked sweet potato
- 4 cups low-sodium vegetable broth
- 1/2 cup diced carrots
- 1/4 cup diced onion
- 1 teaspoon dried thyme
- Salt and pepper to taste

Instructions:
1. In a large saucepan, combine the cooked lentils, diced sweet potato, vegetable broth, carrots, onion, and dried thyme.

2. Bring the mixture to a simmer and cook for 10-15 minutes, or until the carrots and onions are tender.
3. Use an immersion blender or transfer to a regular blender in batches to puree the soup to your desired consistency.
4. Season with salt and pepper to taste.

Chapter 6: DINNER RECIPES

Baked Cod with Lemon Garlic Butter

Ingredients:
- 4 (6 oz) cod fillets
- 2 tablespoons melted butter
- 2 cloves garlic, minced
- 1 tablespoon lemon juice
- Salt and pepper to taste
- Lemon wedges for serving

Instructions:
1. Preheat the oven to 375°F (190°C).
2. Place the cod fillets in a baking dish and season with salt and pepper.

3. In a small bowl, mix together the melted butter, minced garlic, and lemon juice.
4. Pour the lemon garlic butter mixture over the cod fillets, making sure to coat them evenly.
5. Bake for 15-20 minutes, or until the fish is opaque and flakes easily with a fork.
6. Serve hot with lemon wedges on the side.

Meatballs with Marinara Sauce over Mashed Potatoes

Ingredients:
- 1 lb lean ground turkey or beef
- 1 egg
- 1/2 cup breadcrumbs
- 1/4 cup grated Parmesan cheese
- 1 teaspoon dried oregano
- Salt and pepper to taste
- 1 (24 oz) jar low-sodium marinara sauce
- 4 cups prepared mashed potatoes

Instructions:

1. Preheat the oven to 375°F (190°C).
2. In a large bowl, mix together the ground turkey or beef, egg, breadcrumbs, Parmesan cheese, dried oregano, salt, and pepper until well combined.
3. Form the mixture into meatballs, about 1-inch in size.
4. Place the meatballs on a baking sheet and bake for 15-20 minutes, or until cooked through.
5. In a saucepan, heat the marinara sauce over medium heat.
6. Add the baked meatballs to the marinara sauce and simmer for 5-10 minutes, stirring occasionally.
7. Serve the meatballs and sauce over the prepared mashed potatoes.

Vegetable and Tofu Stir-Fry with Rice

Ingredients:

- 1 block (14 oz) firm tofu, drained and cubed

- 2 tablespoons vegetable oil
- 1 cup sliced bell peppers
- 1 cup sliced mushrooms
- 1 cup sliced zucchini
- 1 cup snow peas or sugar snap peas
- 2 cloves garlic, minced
- 2 tablespoons low-sodium soy sauce or tamari
- Cooked white rice or quinoa for serving

Instructions:

1. In a large skillet or wok, heat the vegetable oil over high heat.
2. Add the cubed tofu and stir-fry for 2-3 minutes until lightly browned.
3. Add the sliced bell peppers, mushrooms, zucchini, snow peas or sugar snap peas, and minced garlic to the skillet.
4. Stir-fry for 5-7 minutes, or until the vegetables are tender-crisp.
5. Add the soy sauce or tamari and stir to combine.

6. Serve the vegetable and tofu stir-fry over cooked white rice or quinoa.

Shepherd's Pie with Mashed Cauliflower Topping

Ingredients:
- 1 lb lean ground turkey or beef
- 1 cup diced carrots
- 1 cup diced celery
- 1 cup diced onion
- 1 (14 oz) can low-sodium beef broth
- 2 tablespoons tomato paste
- 1 teaspoon dried thyme
- Salt and pepper to taste
- 4 cups mashed cauliflower (or mashed potatoes)

Instructions:
1. Preheat the oven to 375°F (190°C).
2. In a large skillet, cook the ground turkey or beef over medium-high heat until browned and crumbled. Drain any excess fat.
3. Add the diced carrots, celery, and onion to the skillet and cook for 5-7

minutes, or until the vegetables are tender.

4. Stir in the beef broth, tomato paste, dried thyme, salt, and pepper. Bring the mixture to a simmer and cook for 5 minutes.
5. Transfer the meat and vegetable mixture to a baking dish.
6. Spread the mashed cauliflower (or mashed potatoes) evenly over the top of the meat mixture.
7. Bake for 25-30 minutes, or until the top is lightly browned and the filling is bubbly.

Lemon Garlic Shrimp with Zucchini Noodles

Ingredients:
- 1 lb shrimp, peeled and deveined
- 2 tablespoons olive oil
- 3 cloves garlic, minced
- 1/4 cup lemon juice
- 2 tablespoons butter
- 1/4 cup chopped fresh parsley

- Salt and pepper to taste
- 4 cups zucchini noodles (or cooked pasta)

Instructions:

1. In a large skillet, heat the olive oil over medium-high heat.
2. Add the minced garlic and cook for 1 minute, or until fragrant.
3. Add the shrimp and lemon juice to the skillet. Cook for 3-4 minutes, stirring occasionally, until the shrimp turn opaque.
4. Remove the skillet from heat and stir in the butter and chopped parsley.
5. Season with salt and pepper to taste.
6. Serve the lemon garlic shrimp over zucchini noodles or cooked pasta.

Baked Chicken and Rice Casserole

Ingredients:

- 4 boneless, skinless chicken breasts
- 2 cups cooked white rice
- 1 (10.5 oz) can cream of mushroom soup

- 1/2 cup low-fat milk
- 1/2 cup sliced mushrooms
- 1/4 cup grated Parmesan cheese
- Salt and pepper to taste

Instructions:

1. Preheat the oven to 375°F (190°C).
2. Grease a 9x13 inch baking dish.
3. Place the chicken breasts in the baking dish and season with salt and pepper.
4. In a separate bowl, mix together the cooked rice, cream of mushroom soup, milk, sliced mushrooms, and Parmesan cheese.
5. Spread the rice mixture evenly over the chicken breasts.
6. Cover the baking dish with foil and bake for 45-60 minutes, or until the chicken is cooked through.
7. Remove the foil for the last 10 minutes of baking to allow the top to brown.

Lentil and Sweet Potato Curry

Ingredients:

- 1 cup cooked lentils

- 1 cup diced cooked sweet potato
- 1 (14 oz) can diced tomatoes
- 1 cup coconut milk
- 1 onion, diced
- 2 cloves garlic, minced
- 1 tablespoon curry powder
- 1 teaspoon ground cumin
- Salt and pepper to taste
- Cooked white rice or quinoa for serving

Instructions:

1. In a large saucepan, sauté the diced onion and minced garlic in a little oil or water over medium heat until softened.
2. Add the curry powder and ground cumin, and cook for 1 minute, stirring constantly.
3. Add the cooked lentils, diced sweet potato, diced tomatoes (with juice), and coconut milk to the saucepan.
4. Bring the mixture to a simmer and cook for 10-15 minutes, stirring

occasionally, to allow the flavors to blend.

5. Season with salt and pepper to taste.
6. Serve the lentil and sweet potato curry over cooked white rice or quinoa.

Turkey Meatloaf with Mashed Potatoes

Ingredients:

- 1 lb lean ground turkey
- 1 egg
- 1/2 cup breadcrumbs
- 1/4 cup grated Parmesan cheese
- 1/4 cup low-fat milk
- 1 onion, diced
- 2 cloves garlic, minced
- 1 teaspoon dried thyme
- Salt and pepper to taste
- 4 cups prepared mashed potatoes

Instructions:

1. Preheat the oven to 375°F (190°C).
2. In a large bowl, mix together the ground turkey, egg, breadcrumbs, Parmesan cheese, milk, diced onion,

minced garlic, dried thyme, salt, and pepper until well combined.

3. Transfer the mixture to a loaf pan and shape into a loaf.

4. Bake for 45-60 minutes, or until the meatloaf is cooked through and the internal temperature reaches 165°F (74°C).

5. Let the meatloaf rest for 5-10 minutes before slicing and serving with the prepared mashed potatoes.

Grilled Salmon with Roasted Vegetables

Ingredients:
- 4 (6 oz) salmon fillets
- 2 cups diced potatoes
- 2 cups diced zucchini
- 2 cups diced bell peppers
- 2 tablespoons olive oil
- Salt and pepper to taste
- Lemon wedges for serving

Instructions:
1. Preheat the oven to 400°F (200°C).

2. Toss the diced potatoes, zucchini, and bell peppers with olive oil, salt, and pepper. Spread the vegetables in a single layer on a baking sheet.
3. Roast the vegetables in the preheated oven for 20-25 minutes, or until tender and lightly browned, stirring occasionally.
4. While the vegetables are roasting, preheat a grill or grill pan to medium-high heat.
5. Season the salmon fillets with salt and pepper.
6. Grill the salmon for 4-6 minutes per side, or until it flakes easily with a fork.
7. Serve the grilled salmon with the roasted vegetables and lemon wedges on the side.

Vegetarian Chili

Ingredients:

- 1 (15 oz) can kidney beans, drained and rinsed

- 1 (15 oz) can black beans, drained and rinsed
- 1 (15 oz) can diced tomatoes
- 1 cup diced bell peppers
- 1 cup diced onion
- 2 cloves garlic, minced
- 2 tablespoons chili powder
- 1 teaspoon ground cumin
- Salt and pepper to taste

Instructions:

1. In a large pot or Dutch oven, sauté the diced onion and minced garlic in a little oil or water over medium heat until softened.
2. Add the diced bell peppers and cook for 2-3 minutes.
3. Stir in the diced tomatoes (with juice), kidney beans, black beans, chili powder, and ground cumin.
4. Bring the mixture to a simmer and cook for 15-20 minutes, stirring occasionally, to allow the flavors to blend.
5. Season with salt and pepper to taste.

6. Serve the vegetarian chili hot, garnished with your favorite toppings such as shredded cheese, diced avocado, or sliced green onions.

Baked Tilapia with Lemon and Herbs

Ingredients:
- 4 (6 oz) tilapia fillets
- 2 tablespoons olive oil
- 2 tablespoons lemon juice
- 2 cloves garlic, minced
- 1 teaspoon dried parsley
- 1 teaspoon dried thyme
- Salt and pepper to taste
- Lemon wedges for serving

Instructions:
1. Preheat the oven to 400°F (200°C).
2. Rinse the tilapia fillets and pat them dry with paper towels.
3. In a small bowl, combine the olive oil, lemon juice, minced garlic, dried parsley, dried thyme, salt, and pepper.

4. Place the tilapia fillets in a baking dish and pour the lemon-herb mixture over the top, making sure to coat the fillets evenly.
5. Bake for 12-15 minutes, or until the fish is opaque and flakes easily with a fork.
6. Serve hot with lemon wedges on the side.

Shrimp Scampi

Ingredients:
- 1 lb large shrimp, peeled and deveined
- 3 tablespoons butter
- 2 cloves garlic, minced
- 2 tablespoons lemon juice
- 2 tablespoons chopped fresh parsley
- Salt and pepper to taste
- Cooked white rice or pasta for serving (optional)

Instructions:
1. In a large skillet, melt the butter over medium-high heat.

2. Add the minced garlic and cook for 1 minute, or until fragrant.
3. Add the shrimp to the skillet and cook for 2-3 minutes, stirring occasionally, until they start to turn pink.
4. Add the lemon juice, chopped parsley, salt, and pepper. Stir to combine.
5. Cook for an additional 2-3 minutes, or until the shrimp are fully cooked through.
6. Serve the shrimp scampi hot, over cooked white rice or pasta if desired.

Tuna Salad

Ingredients:
- 2 (5 oz) cans tuna, drained
- 1/4 cup low-fat mayonnaise
- 2 tablespoons diced celery
- 2 tablespoons diced red onion (optional)
- 1 tablespoon lemon juice
- Salt and pepper to taste
- Lettuce leaves for serving

Instructions:

1. In a medium bowl, flake the drained tuna with a fork.
2. Add the low-fat mayonnaise, diced celery, diced red onion (if using), lemon juice, salt, and pepper.
3. Mix well until all ingredients are combined.
4. Serve the tuna salad on lettuce leaves or on top of a bed of greens.

Salmon Patties

Ingredients:
- 1 (14.75 oz) can salmon, drained and flaked
- 1 egg, beaten
- 1/4 cup breadcrumbs
- 2 tablespoons diced onion
- 2 tablespoons chopped fresh parsley
- 1 tablespoon lemon juice
- Salt and pepper to taste
- 2 tablespoons olive oil for cooking

Instructions:
1. In a bowl, combine the drained and flaked salmon, beaten egg,

breadcrumbs, diced onion, chopped parsley, lemon juice, salt, and pepper. Mix well.

2. Form the mixture into patties, about 1/2 inch thick.
3. Heat the olive oil in a large skillet over medium heat.
4. Cook the salmon patties for 3-4 minutes per side, or until golden brown and cooked through.
5. Serve hot, with lemon wedges on the side if desired.

Cod with Tomato and Herb Sauce

Ingredients:
- 4 (6 oz) cod fillets
- 2 tablespoons olive oil
- 1 onion, diced
- 2 cloves garlic, minced
- 1 (14.5 oz) can diced tomatoes
- 1 teaspoon dried oregano
- 1 teaspoon dried basil
- Salt and pepper to taste
- Chopped fresh parsley for garnish

Instructions:

1. In a large skillet, heat the olive oil over medium heat.
2. Add the diced onion and minced garlic, and cook for 2-3 minutes, or until the onion is translucent.
3. Add the diced tomatoes (with juice), dried oregano, dried basil, salt, and pepper. Stir to combine.
4. Nestle the cod fillets into the tomato sauce, spooning some of the sauce over the top of the fish.
5. Cover the skillet and simmer for 10-12 minutes, or until the fish is opaque and flakes easily with a fork.
6. Garnish with chopped fresh parsley before serving.

Baked Cod with Breadcrumb Topping

Ingredients:

- 4 (6 oz) cod fillets
- 1/2 cup breadcrumbs
- 2 tablespoons grated Parmesan cheese
- 2 tablespoons melted butter

- 1 teaspoon dried parsley
- 1 teaspoon lemon zest
- Salt and pepper to taste
- Lemon wedges for serving

Instructions:

1. Preheat the oven to 400°F (200°C).
2. Rinse the cod fillets and pat them dry with paper towels. Place them in a baking dish.
3. In a small bowl, combine the breadcrumbs, Parmesan cheese, melted butter, dried parsley, lemon zest, salt, and pepper.
4. Evenly sprinkle the breadcrumb mixture over the top of the cod fillets, pressing gently to adhere.
5. Bake for 12-15 minutes, or until the fish is opaque and flakes easily with a fork.
6. Serve hot with lemon wedges on the side.

Shrimp and Vegetable Skewers

Ingredients:

- 1 lb large shrimp, peeled and deveined
- 1 zucchini, cut into 1-inch pieces
- 1 red bell pepper, cut into 1-inch pieces
- 1 red onion, cut into wedges
- 2 tablespoons olive oil
- 1 teaspoon dried oregano
- Salt and pepper to taste
- Lemon wedges for serving

Instructions:

1. Preheat the grill or grill pan to medium-high heat.
2. Thread the shrimp, zucchini, bell pepper, and red onion onto skewers, alternating between the different ingredients.
3. In a small bowl, combine the olive oil, dried oregano, salt, and pepper.
4. Brush the skewers with the olive oil mixture, coating them evenly.
5. Grill the skewers for 8-10 minutes, turning occasionally, until the shrimp are opaque and the vegetables are tender.

6. Serve hot with lemon wedges on the side.

Tuna Melt Sandwiches

Ingredients:
- 2 (5 oz) cans tuna, drained
- 1/4 cup low-fat mayonnaise
- 2 tablespoons diced celery
- 1 tablespoon diced red onion (optional)
- Salt and pepper to taste
- 4 slices white or sourdough bread
- 4 slices low-fat cheddar cheese

Instructions:
1. In a bowl, flake the drained tuna with a fork.
2. Add the low-fat mayonnaise, diced celery, diced red onion (if using), salt, and pepper. Mix well.
3. Toast the bread slices.
4. Spread the tuna mixture evenly onto two slices of bread.
5. Top each sandwich with two slices of cheddar cheese.

6. Place the sandwiches on a baking sheet and broil for 2-3 minutes, or until the cheese is melted and bubbly.

Shrimp and Vegetable Fried Rice

Ingredients:
- 1 lb shrimp, peeled and deveined
- 2 cups cooked white rice
- 1 cup diced carrots
- 1 cup diced bell peppers
- 1/2 cup diced onion
- 2 cloves garlic, minced
- 2 eggs, beaten
- 2 tablespoons low-sodium soy sauce
- 2 tablespoons vegetable oil

Instructions:
1. Heat the vegetable oil in a large skillet or wok over high heat.
2. Add the shrimp and cook for 2-3 minutes, or until they start to turn pink. Remove the shrimp from the skillet and set aside.

3. In the same skillet, scramble the beaten eggs and remove them from the skillet once cooked.
4. Add the diced carrots, bell peppers, onion, and minced garlic to the skillet. Stir-fry for 2-3 minutes.
5. Add the cooked rice, soy sauce, cooked shrimp, and scrambled eggs to the skillet. Stir-fry for an additional 2-3 minutes, or until everything is heated through and well combined.

Crab Cakes

Ingredients:
- 1 (6 oz) can lump crabmeat, drained and flaked
- 1/4 cup breadcrumbs
- 1 egg, beaten
- 2 tablespoons low-fat mayonnaise
- 1 tablespoon Dijon mustard
- 1 tablespoon chopped fresh parsley
- 1 teaspoon lemon juice
- Salt and pepper to taste
- 2 tablespoons olive oil for cooking

Instructions:

1. In a bowl, combine the drained and flaked crabmeat, breadcrumbs, beaten egg, low-fat mayonnaise, Dijon mustard, chopped parsley, lemon juice, salt, and pepper. Mix well.
2. Form the mixture into patties, about 1/2 inch thick.
3. Heat the olive oil in a large skillet over medium heat.
4. Cook the crab cakes for 3-4 minutes per side, or until golden brown and cooked through.
5. Serve hot, with lemon wedges or tartar sauce on the side, if desired.

Chapter 8: SNACKS RECIPES

Baked Banana Chips

Ingredients:

- 2 ripe bananas, thinly sliced
- 1 tablespoon lemon juice
- 1 tablespoon honey (optional)

- 1/4 teaspoon ground cinnamon (optional)

Instructions:

1. Preheat the oven to 250°F (120°C).
2. Line a baking sheet with parchment paper.
3. In a bowl, toss the thinly sliced bananas with lemon juice, honey (if using), and ground cinnamon (if using).
4. Arrange the banana slices in a single layer on the prepared baking sheet.
5. Bake for 1 to 1 1/2 hours, flipping the banana slices halfway through, until they are dried and crispy.
6. Let the banana chips cool completely before serving.

Avocado Toast

Ingredients:

- 2 slices of white or sourdough bread
- 1 ripe avocado, mashed
- 1 teaspoon lemon juice
- Salt and pepper to taste

- Optional toppings: sliced tomatoes, sliced cucumbers, or a sprinkle of dried herbs

Instructions:

1. Toast the bread slices.
2. In a small bowl, mash the avocado with lemon juice, salt, and pepper.
3. Spread the mashed avocado mixture evenly onto the toasted bread slices.
4. Top with sliced tomatoes, sliced cucumbers, or a sprinkle of dried herbs, if desired.

Yogurt Parfait

Ingredients:

- 1 cup low-fat plain yogurt
- 1/2 cup diced peaches or strawberries (fresh or canned in water)
- 2 tablespoons low-fat granola or crushed graham crackers

Instructions:

1. In a small bowl or parfait glass, layer half of the yogurt, then half of the diced fruit.

2. Sprinkle with half of the granola or crushed graham crackers.
3. Repeat the layers with the remaining yogurt, fruit, and granola or crushed graham crackers.
4. Serve chilled.

Hummus and Vegetable Sticks

Ingredients:
- 1 cup hummus (store-bought or homemade)
- 1 cucumber, cut into sticks
- 1 bell pepper, cut into strips
- 1 carrot, cut into sticks

Instructions:
1. Arrange the hummus in a small serving bowl.
2. Arrange the cucumber, bell pepper, and carrot sticks on a plate or platter around the hummus.
3. Serve the hummus and vegetables together for dipping.

Smoothie Bowl

Ingredients:

- 1 cup low-fat milk or non-dairy milk
- 1 banana
- 1/2 cup frozen berries
- 1 tablespoon honey or maple syrup (optional)
- Toppings: sliced bananas, granola, chia seeds, or chopped nuts

Instructions:

1. In a blender, combine the milk, banana, frozen berries, and honey or maple syrup (if using).
2. Blend until smooth and creamy.
3. Pour the smoothie mixture into a bowl.
4. Top with sliced bananas, granola, chia seeds, or chopped nuts.
5. Serve immediately.

Chapter 9: DESSERT RECIPES

Rice Pudding

Ingredients:

- 1 cup cooked white rice
- 2 cups low-fat milk
- 1/4 cup sugar
- 1 teaspoon vanilla extract
- 1/4 teaspoon ground cinnamon
- 1/4 cup raisins (optional)

Instructions:

1. In a saucepan, combine the cooked rice, milk, sugar, and vanilla extract.
2. Bring the mixture to a simmer over medium heat, stirring frequently.
3. Reduce the heat to low and cook for 15-20 minutes, stirring occasionally, until the mixture thickens to your desired consistency.
4. Remove from heat and stir in the ground cinnamon and raisins (if using).
5. Serve warm or chilled.

Baked Apples

Ingredients:

- 4 medium apples
- 1/4 cup brown sugar

- 1/4 cup water
- 1 teaspoon ground cinnamon
- 2 tablespoons butter or margarine

Instructions:

1. Preheat the oven to 375°F (190°C).
2. Core the apples, leaving the bottom intact, and place them in a baking dish.
3. In a small bowl, mix together the brown sugar, water, and ground cinnamon.
4. Fill the cored apples with the brown sugar mixture.
5. Top each apple with a small pat of butter or margarine.
6. Bake for 30-40 minutes, or until the apples are tender when pierced with a fork.
7. Serve warm, with the syrup from the baking dish spooned over the top.

Fruit Salad

Ingredients:

- 1 cup diced pineapple

- 1 cup diced peaches or pears (fresh or canned in water)
- 1 cup diced mango or papaya
- 1 cup diced strawberries or grapes
- 2 tablespoons honey or maple syrup (optional)
- 1 tablespoon lemon juice (optional)

Instructions:

1. In a large bowl, combine the diced pineapple, peaches or pears, mango or papaya, and strawberries or grapes.
2. Drizzle with honey or maple syrup (if desired) and lemon juice (if desired).
3. Gently toss the fruit salad to coat the fruit with the dressing.
4. Refrigerate for at least 30 minutes before serving to allow the flavors to blend.

Banana Bread

Ingredients:

- 1 3/4 cups all-purpose flour
- 1 teaspoon baking soda
- 1/4 teaspoon salt

- 1/2 cup sugar
- 1/4 cup unsweetened applesauce
- 1/4 cup low-fat milk or non-dairy milk
- 2 ripe bananas, mashed
- 1 egg
- 1 teaspoon vanilla extract

Instructions:

1. Preheat the oven to 350°F (175°C).
2. In a large bowl, whisk together the flour, baking soda, salt, and sugar.
3. In a separate bowl, mix together the applesauce, milk, mashed bananas, egg, and vanilla extract.
4. Add the wet ingredients to the dry ingredients and stir until just combined (do not overmix).
5. Pour the batter into a greased loaf pan.
6. Bake for 50-60 minutes, or until a toothpick inserted into the center comes out clean.
7. Let the banana bread cool in the pan for 10 minutes before removing and slicing.

Peanut Butter Cookies

Ingredients:

- 1 cup creamy peanut butter
- 1 cup sugar
- 1 egg
- 1 teaspoon baking soda
- 1/2 teaspoon vanilla extract

Instructions:

1. Preheat the oven to 350°F (175°C).
2. In a large bowl, mix together the peanut butter and sugar until well combined.
3. Add the egg, baking soda, and vanilla extract to the peanut butter mixture and mix until fully incorporated.
4. Roll the dough into small balls, about 1-inch in size, and place them on a baking sheet lined with parchment paper, spacing them about 2 inches apart.
5. Use a fork to gently press down on each dough ball, creating a criss-cross pattern on the top.

6. Bake for 8-10 minutes, or until lightly golden brown.

7. Let the cookies cool on the baking sheet for a few minutes before transferring them to a wire rack to cool completely.

Chapter 10: BEVERAGES RECIPES

Fruit Smoothie

Ingredients:

- 1 cup low-fat milk or non-dairy milk
- 1 banana
- 1/2 cup frozen berries (e.g., strawberries, blueberries, raspberries)
- 1 tablespoon honey or maple syrup (optional)

Instructions:

1. Add the milk, banana, frozen berries, and honey or maple syrup (if using) to a blender.

2. Blend until smooth and creamy.

3. Serve immediately or chill in the refrigerator before serving.

4. Lemon-Ginger   Infused   Water
Ingredients:

- 1 lemon, sliced
- 2-inch piece of fresh ginger, thinly sliced
- 4 cups water

Instructions:

1. In a large pitcher or container, combine the sliced lemon, sliced ginger, and water.
2. Refrigerate for at least 2 hours to allow the flavors to infuse.
3. Serve chilled and enjoy the refreshing lemon-ginger taste.

Iced Herbal Tea

Ingredients:

- 4 herbal tea bags (e.g., chamomile, peppermint, or hibiscus)
- 4 cups water
- Honey or lemon slices (optional)

Instructions:

1. Bring the water to a boil in a saucepan or kettle.

2. Remove from heat and add the herbal tea bags. Steep for 5-7 minutes.
3. Remove the tea bags and let the tea cool to room temperature.
4. Transfer the tea to a pitcher and refrigerate until chilled.
5. Serve over ice and add honey or lemon slices, if desired.

Golden Milk (Turmeric Latte)

Ingredients:
- 2 cups low-fat milk or non-dairy milk
- 1 teaspoon ground turmeric
- 1/2 teaspoon ground cinnamon
- 1/4 teaspoon ground ginger
- 1 tablespoon honey or maple syrup (optional)

Instructions:
1. In a small saucepan, whisk together the milk, turmeric, cinnamon, and ginger.
2. Heat the mixture over medium heat, whisking frequently, until it starts to

steam and bubble around the edges (do not boil).

3. Remove from heat and stir in the honey or maple syrup, if desired.

4. Pour the golden milk into mugs and serve warm.

Cucumber-Mint Infused Water

Ingredients:

- 1 cucumber, thinly sliced
- 10-12 fresh mint leaves
- 4 cups water

Instructions:

1. In a large pitcher or container, combine the sliced cucumber, mint leaves, and water.

2. Refrigerate for at least 2 hours to allow the flavors to infuse.

3. Serve chilled and enjoy the refreshing cucumber-mint taste.

Cucumber Bites

Ingredients:
- 1 large cucumber
- 1 cup low-fat cream cheese or plain Greek yogurt
- 1/4 cup finely chopped fresh dill or chives
- Salt and pepper to taste

Instructions:
1. Slice the cucumber into 1/2-inch thick rounds.
2. In a small bowl, mix together the cream cheese or yogurt, chopped dill or chives, and salt and pepper.
3. Spread a small amount of the cream cheese or yogurt mixture onto each cucumber slice.
4. Refrigerate for at least 30 minutes before serving to allow the flavors to blend.

Caprese Skewers

Ingredients:

- 1 pint cherry tomatoes
- 8 oz fresh mozzarella cheese, cut into small cubes
- Fresh basil leaves
- Balsamic glaze or balsamic vinegar (optional)
- Wooden skewers

Instructions:

1. Thread the cherry tomatoes, mozzarella cubes, and basil leaves onto the wooden skewers, alternating the ingredients.
2. Drizzle with balsamic glaze or balsamic vinegar (if using).
3. Serve chilled or at room temperature.

Deviled Eggs

Ingredients:

- 6 hard-boiled eggs
- 1/4 cup low-fat mayonnaise
- 1 teaspoon Dijon mustard

- 1 tablespoon finely chopped fresh parsley
- Salt and pepper to taste
- Paprika for garnish (optional)

Instructions:

1. Peel the hard-boiled eggs and cut them in half lengthwise.
2. Remove the yolks and place them in a small bowl.
3. Mash the yolks with a fork and mix in the mayonnaise, Dijon mustard, chopped parsley, salt, and pepper.
4. Spoon or pipe the yolk mixture back into the egg white halves.
5. Sprinkle with paprika for garnish (if desired).
6. Refrigerate until ready to serve.

Hummus with Vegetable Sticks

Ingredients:

- 1 cup hummus (store-bought or homemade)
- 1 cucumber, cut into sticks
- 1 carrot, cut into sticks

- 1 bell pepper, cut into strips
- 1 zucchini, cut into sticks

Instructions:

1. Arrange the hummus in a small serving bowl.
2. Arrange the cucumber, carrot, bell pepper, and zucchini sticks on a plate or platter around the hummus.
3. Serve the hummus and vegetables together for dipping.

Fruit Skewers with Yogurt Dip

Ingredients:

- 1 cup fresh fruits (e.g., strawberries, grapes, melon, pineapple, kiwi)
- 1 cup low-fat plain Greek yogurt
- 1 tablespoon honey
- 1/2 teaspoon vanilla extract
- Wooden skewers

Instructions:

1. Thread the fresh fruit onto the wooden skewers, alternating different types of fruit.

2. In a small bowl, mix together the yogurt, honey, and vanilla extract.
3. Serve the fruit skewers with the yogurt dip on the side.

Roasted Sweet Potato Rounds

Ingredients:
- 2 medium sweet potatoes, sliced into 1/4-inch rounds
- 2 tablespoons olive oil
- 1 teaspoon paprika
- Salt and pepper to taste

Instructions:
1. Preheat the oven to 400°F (200°C).
2. In a large bowl, toss the sweet potato rounds with olive oil, paprika, salt, and pepper until evenly coated.
3. Arrange the sweet potato rounds in a single layer on a baking sheet.
4. Roast for 20-25 minutes, flipping halfway, until tender and lightly browned.
5. Serve warm or at room temperature.

Avocado Toast Bites

Ingredients:
- 1 ripe avocado, mashed
- 1 tablespoon lemon juice
- 1 loaf of white or sourdough bread, sliced and cut into bite-sized squares
- Salt and pepper to taste
- Optional toppings: diced tomatoes, sliced cucumbers, or red pepper flakes

Instructions:
1. In a small bowl, mash the avocado with lemon juice, salt, and pepper.
2. Toast the bread squares lightly.
3. Spread a small amount of the mashed avocado mixture onto each toast square.
4. Top with diced tomatoes, sliced cucumbers, or red pepper flakes (if desired).

Baked Zucchini Fries

Ingredients:
- 2 medium zucchinis, cut into 1/4-inch thick sticks

- 1 egg white, beaten
- 1/2 cup breadcrumbs
- 1/4 cup grated Parmesan cheese
- 1 teaspoon dried Italian seasoning
- Salt and pepper to taste

Instructions:

1. Preheat the oven to 400°F (200°C).
2. In a shallow bowl, beat the egg white.
3. In another shallow bowl, mix together the breadcrumbs, Parmesan cheese, Italian seasoning, salt, and pepper.
4. Dip the zucchini sticks into the egg white, then coat them with the breadcrumb mixture.
5. Arrange the coated zucchini sticks on a baking sheet in a single layer.
6. Bake for 15-20 minutes, or until golden brown and crispy.
7. Serve warm with a dipping sauce of your choice.

Tomato Basil Bruschetta

Ingredients:

- 4 Roma tomatoes, diced

- 1/4 cup diced red onion
- 2 tablespoons chopped fresh basil
- 2 tablespoons olive oil
- 1 tablespoon balsamic vinegar
- Salt and pepper to taste
- 1 baguette, sliced into 1/2-inch rounds and toasted

Instructions:

1. In a bowl, combine the diced tomatoes, red onion, chopped basil, olive oil, balsamic vinegar, salt, and pepper. Mix well.
2. Spoon the tomato mixture onto the toasted baguette rounds.
3. Serve immediately or let the flavors marinate for 30 minutes before serving.

Stuffed Mushroom Caps

Ingredients:

- 12 large mushroom caps
- 1/2 cup breadcrumbs
- 1/4 cup grated Parmesan cheese
- 2 tablespoons chopped fresh parsley

- 2 cloves garlic, minced
- 2 tablespoons olive oil
- Salt and pepper to taste

Instructions:

1. Preheat the oven to 375°F (190°C).
2. Remove the stems from the mushroom caps and finely chop the stems.
3. In a bowl, mix together the chopped mushroom stems, breadcrumbs, Parmesan cheese, parsley, garlic, olive oil, salt, and pepper.
4. Spoon the filling mixture into the mushroom caps, pressing gently to fill the caps.
5. Arrange the stuffed mushroom caps on a baking sheet.
6. Bake for 15-20 minutes, or until the filling is golden brown and the mushrooms are tender.
7. Serve warm.

CONCLUSION

"Taking the first step towards understanding and managing your ostomy can be daunting, but with the right guidance, you can regain control and confidence in your life. Our Colostomy, Ileostomy, and Ostomy Program for Beginners is the ultimate resource for those starting their ostomy journey. With our comprehensive and easy-to-follow guide, you'll learn how to navigate the physical and emotional aspects of ostomy care, regain your independence, and live a full and active life. Empower yourself with knowledge and take the first step towards a happier, healthier you. Get your copy today!"

THE END